Men's Guide to Multi-Orgasmic Sex

A Comprehensive Guide for Men to Achieving Multi-Orgasmic Sex, Mastering Pleasure, and Embracing Sexual Empowerment for Lifelong Fulfillment and Intimate Connection

Cheryl Bach

Men's Guide to Multi-Orgasmic Sex

Cheryl Bach

Table of Contents

Introduction

Sexual pleasure is a crucial aspect of human life. It is one commonality that exists in all relationships, whether romantic or otherwise. The feeling of connection, pleasure, and fulfillment that comes from sexual encounters is what makes such experiences worthwhile. However, men are often overlooked when it comes to achieving multiple orgasms during sex. This book aims to provide a comprehensive guide for men to achieving multi-orgasmic sex, mastering pleasure, and embracing sexual empowerment for lifelong fulfillment and intimate connection.

Multi-orgasmic sex is the ability to experience successive orgasms in a single sexual encounter. While this may seem like an impossible feat for some men, it is achievable with the right tools and knowledge. Multi-orgasmic sex is not only an indicator of sexual prowess but also an essential aspect of men's sexual health and wellness.

The Benefits of Mastering Multi-Orgasmic Sex

Men who can master multi-orgasmic sex enjoy numerous benefits that contribute to their overall well-being, including intimacy, connection, and fulfillment. The ability to achieve multiple orgasms can lead to longer, more intense, and enjoyable sexual experiences, which can improve the quality of relationships and sexual encounters.

The Purpose of the Book and What to Expect

The purpose of this book is to provide a comprehensive guide to men who wish to embrace sexual empowerment by achieving multi-orgasmic sex. The book comprises practical advice, tips, and exercises to help men improve their sexual health, wellness, and performance in the bedroom. The chapters in this book will provide an in-depth understanding of multi-orgasmic sex, including the steps to achieving it, the benefits of practicing it, and how to embrace sexual empowerment.

The book will also include detailed information on techniques such as tantric sex, kegel exercises, and edging that men can use to achieve multi-orgasmic sex. Additionally, it will address common myths about male sexuality and empower men to take control of their sexual experiences.

In conclusion, this book is an essential guide for every man who wants to achieve multi-orgasmic sex, master pleasure, and embrace sexual empowerment for lifelong fulfillment and intimate connection. The chapters in this book will provide practical tips, tools, and techniques that can help men achieve their goals while also promoting their overall sexual health and wellness.

Chapter 1

Understanding Male Sexual Anatomy and Response

In order to achieve multi-orgasmic sex and master pleasure, it is crucial for men to understand their sexual anatomy and how it works. This knowledge allows men to identify the different stages of the sexual response cycle and make adjustments that can heighten their sexual pleasure.

Male Anatomy

The male reproductive system is composed of internal and external structures that work together to facilitate sexual function and reproduction. The external organs include the penis, scrotum, and testicles, while the internal structures include the vas deferens, prostate gland, seminal vesicles, and urethra. The penis is the primary organ involved in sexual intercourse and is composed of three parts: the root, shaft, and glans. The shaft contains the corpora cavernosa and corpus spongiosum, which fill with blood during an erection.

How the Male Sexual Response Works

The male sexual response cycle is a complex process that involves physical and psychological stimuli. It can be divided into four stages: excitement, plateau, orgasm, and resolution. During the excitement phase, physical and mental arousal occurs, leading to an increase in blood flow to the penis, resulting in an erection. In the plateau phase, sexual arousal is heightened, and the body prepares for orgasm. During the orgasm phase, there is a release of sexual tension, resulting in rhythmic muscular contractions in the genital region and ejaculation. Finally, the resolution phase involves a decrease in sexual tension, leading to a return to a pre-aroused state.

Cheryl Bach

Common Misconceptions about Male Orgasms

One common misconception about male orgasms is that they are solely achieved through penile stimulation. However, research has shown that orgasm can also occur through the stimulation of other parts of the body, such as the nipples and prostate gland. Another misconception is that men have a harder time achieving multiple orgasms than women, but with the right techniques and practice, men can learn to achieve multiple orgasms just as easily as women.

The Role of the Mind-Body Connection in Sexual Pleasure

Sexual pleasure is not only a physical experience but also involves a strong mind-body connection. Mental factors such as anxiety, stress, and self-consciousness can interfere with sexual pleasure. On the other hand, positive emotions such as relaxation, confidence, and trust in one's partner can enhance sexual pleasure. By mastering mindfulness and focusing on the present moment during sexual encounters, men can improve their ability to achieve multiple orgasms.

In conclusion, understanding male sexual anatomy and response is crucial for men who want to master pleasure and achieve multi-orgasmic sex. Men who take the time to learn about their bodies and how they respond to different stimuli can improve their sexual experiences in numerous ways. By understanding their anatomy, men can identify the areas that are most sensitive to touch and develop techniques that enhance sexual pleasure. Knowing the different stages of the sexual response cycle can also help men prolong sexual encounters and achieve multiple orgasms.

It is important to note that sexual pleasure is not solely a physical experience and involves a strong mind-body connection. By maintaining a relaxed and focused state of mind during sexual activity, men can heighten their pleasure and improve their ability to achieve multiple orgasms.

Chapter 2

Preparing Your Mind and Body for Multi-Orgasmic Sex

The ability to achieve multiple orgasms is not solely dependent on physical technique and prowess. Preparing the mind and body for sexual experiences is just as crucial in achieving multi-orgasmic sex. In this chapter, we will explore the importance of relaxation, mental focus, breathing techniques, meditation practices, physical exercise, and healthy eating habits to enhance sexual energy and stamina.

The Importance of Relaxation and Mental Focus for Achieving Multiple Orgasms

Relaxation and mental focus play a significant role in enhancing sexual pleasure. By reducing stress, anxiety, and self-consciousness, men can increase their ability to focus on their bodies and sexual sensations, leading to more prolonged and pleasurable sexual experiences. Techniques such as deep breathing, visualization, and progressive muscle relaxation can help men achieve this level of relaxation and mental focus.

Breathing Techniques and Meditation Practices to Enhance Sexual Energy and Focus

Breathwork and meditation practices are widely recognized for their ability to increase relaxation, reduce stress, and improve focus. These practices can also enhance sexual energy and pleasure by increasing blood flow to the genitals and improving body awareness. One important technique is deep belly breathing, which involves inhaling deeply through the nose and exhaling through the mouth, allowing the abdomen to expand and contract with each breath. Meditation practices, such as mindfulness meditation, can also help men improve their ability to focus on sexual sensations, leading to more pleasurable experiences.

Physical Exercise and Healthy Eating Habits for Sexual Vitality and Stamina

Physical exercise and healthy eating habits are essential for overall health and vitality, including sexual health. Exercise increases blood flow to the genitals, improves cardiovascular health, and increases stamina, leading to more pleasurable and prolonged sexual experiences. Recommended exercises include pelvic floor exercises and yoga, which can improve pelvic health and increase sexual pleasure.

Incorporating healthy eating habits can also improve sexual vitality and stamina. A diet that is rich in whole foods such as fruits, vegetables, lean proteins, and healthy fats can improve blood flow, reduce inflammation, and enhance hormone production, leading to improved sexual health.

Additionally, consuming foods rich in zinc, such as oysters and almonds, can enhance male sexual function.

In conclusion, preparing the mind and body for sexual experiences is integral to achieving multi-orgasmic sex and mastering sexual pleasure. By incorporating techniques such as relaxation, mental focus, breathing techniques, meditation practices, physical exercise, and healthy eating habits, men can enhance their sexual experience and achieve lifelong fulfillment and intimate connection. The next chapter will explore physical techniques and exercises that can be used to achieve multiple orgasms and increase sexual pleasure.

But before we delve into those techniques, it is important to note that the mind and body are interconnected, and sexual pleasure is not only a physical experience but also a mental one. Therefore, men should take the time to focus on their mental and emotional wellbeing, as this can greatly influence their sexual experiences.

By reducing stress, anxiety, and self-consciousness, men can improve their ability to focus on their bodies and increase sexual sensations, leading to more prolonged and pleasurable experiences. Breathing techniques, meditation practices, physical exercise, and healthy eating habits are all excellent ways to improve mental focus and enhance sexual energy and stamina.

Incorporating these practices into daily life can help men achieve lifelong sexual fulfillment and connection. Men who take the time to prepare their minds and bodies for sexual experiences will find that achieving multiple orgasms and experiencing heightened pleasure becomes easier with time and can be a source of great fulfillment and connection in their lives.

Furthermore, it is important to remember that sexual experiences are unique to each individual, and there is no one-size-fits-all approach to achieving multi-orgasmic sex. Therefore, it is essential for men to experiment with different techniques and find what works best for them.

In summary, preparing the mind and body for sexual experiences is an integral part of achieving multi-orgasmic sex. By incorporating relaxation, mental focus, breathing techniques, meditation practices, physical exercise, and healthy eating habits into daily life, men can enhance their sexual experiences and achieve lifelong fulfillment and intimate connection. The next chapter will explore physical techniques and exercises that can be used to achieve multiple orgasms and increase sexual pleasure.

Chapter 3

Techniques for Building Sexual Energy and Arousal

Achieving multi-orgasmic sex is not only about physical technique, but also about building and channeling sexual energy. In this chapter, we will explore strategies for building sexual energy, the role of foreplay in multi-orgasmic sex, and different techniques for heightening sexual arousal.

Strategies for Building and Channeling Sexual Energy

Building sexual energy involves increasing the flow of blood and energy to the genitals and retaining that energy through various techniques. One strategy is the "squeeze technique," which involves squeezing the base of the penis to prevent ejaculation. Another technique is breathing exercises, which can enhance blood flow and increase sexual energy.

Tantric practices, such as the "microcosmic orbit," are also effective at building and channeling sexual energy. This involves circulating sexual energy throughout the body, focusing on the genitals, and then moving it up and down the spine in a circular motion. This technique can be done alone or with a partner and can help men achieve prolonged and intense sexual pleasure.

The Role of Foreplay in Multi-Orgasmic Sex

Foreplay plays a critical role in multi-orgasmic sex as it helps build excitement, arousal, and anticipation. It is essential to include ample foreplay in sexual experiences to ensure that both partners are fully aroused and ready for more extended and fulfilling sexual experiences.

Foreplay can involve kissing, touching, massaging, or any other activity that builds sexual tension. It is essential to explore different techniques during foreplay and find out what works best for both partners.

Different Techniques for Heightening Sexual Arousal

There are numerous techniques that men can use to heighten their sexual arousal and increase their chances of achieving multiple orgasms. One technique is massage, which can help relax muscles, reduce stress, and increase blood flow to the genitals. It can be done alone or with a partner and can involve using essential oils, candles, or other aromatherapy techniques to enhance the experience.

Kissing is another effective technique for increasing sexual arousal. It can be used as part of foreplay or during sexual intercourse and can involve a variety of techniques, such as light touches, biting, or neck kisses. Kissing can help build intimacy, enhance pleasure, and facilitate deeper connections between partners.

Oral sex is also an effective technique for increasing sexual arousal and pleasure. It can involve giving or receiving oral stimulation, and provides intense sensations that can lead to powerful orgasms. Oral sex should always be done with consent and with a partner who has been tested for sexually transmitted infections.

In conclusion, achieving multi-orgasmic sex requires more than just physical technique. Building and channeling sexual energy, embracing foreplay, and using different techniques to heighten sexual arousal are all critical components of achieving sexual empowerment and lifelong fulfillment. By focusing on both the physical and emotional aspects of sex, men can enhance their sexual experiences and build deeper connections with their partners. The next chapter will explore different positions and techniques that can be used during sexual intercourse to achieve multiple orgasms and increase sexual pleasure.

Chapter 4

The Art of Extended Orgasms

In this chapter, we will explore techniques for extending and intensifying male orgasms, the use of kegel exercises and other body techniques for enhancing pleasure, and exploring edging as a way of building sensation and achieving prolonged pleasure.

Techniques for Extending and Intensifying Male Orgasms

Men can extend and intensify their orgasms through various techniques that enhance their ability to feel and control their bodies. One technique involves using the pubococcygeus (PC) muscle, which controls urine flow and is located between the anus and testicles. By strengthening and contracting this muscle during sexual activity, men can experience longer and more intense orgasms.

Another technique for extending and intensifying orgasms is called the "stop-start" method. This involves stopping sexual stimulation just before ejaculation, waiting for a few seconds, and then resuming stimulation. This technique can help men build up sexual tension, prolong pleasure, and ultimately lead to more powerful orgasms.

The Use of Kegel Exercises and Other Body Techniques for Enhancing Pleasure

Kegel exercises, which involve contracting the PC muscle repeatedly, can not only help to extend and intensify orgasms but can also increase sexual pleasure. By strengthening this muscle, men can have more control over their ejaculation, leading to more extended and fulfilling sexual experiences.

Other body techniques, such as deep breathing, can also help enhance pleasure during sexual activity. By focusing on deep, rhythmic breaths, men can relax and become more attuned to their bodies, allowing them to experience heightened sensations and achieve more intense orgasms.

Exploring Edging as a Way of Building Sensation and Achieving Prolonged Pleasure

Edging is a popular technique that involves bringing yourself or your partner close to orgasm, then backing off, and repeating the process over an extended period. This technique can help build sexual tension, prolong pleasure, and lead to more powerful orgasms.

During edging, it's essential to pay attention to your body's signals and learn to recognize when you're getting close to ejaculation. By slowing down or stopping stimulation before reaching the point of no return, you can prolong the sexual experience and intensify the orgasm when it finally occurs.

There are different approaches to edging, such as experimenting with different techniques and positions, using breathing exercises to calm the mind and body, and incorporating sex toys, pornography, or erotic materials to enhance arousal.

One way to start edging is by practicing solo. Find a comfortable and private space where you can focus on your body and explore your responses to different levels of stimulation. Experiment with different techniques and explore your body's unique responses to different types of touch and pressure. Pay attention to the sensations in your body and learn to recognize when you're close to orgasm. When you feel yourself getting close, slow down or change the intensity of stimulation until you feel in control again.

If you're practicing edging with a partner, communication is key. Let them know what feels good and what doesn't, and how close you are to orgasm. While edging can be a pleasurable experience for both partners, it's essential to respect each other's boundaries, communicate openly, and prioritize each other's pleasure.

It's important to note that edging isn't for everyone, and some people may find it frustrating or unfulfilling. If you're not enjoying the experience, there's no reason to continue. Remember that exploring your sexuality is a personal journey, and it's important to respect your own boundaries and desires.

In conclusion, the art of extended orgasms involves exploring techniques that can help men prolong pleasure, intensify orgasms, and achieve deeper levels of sexual fulfillment. By focusing on both physical and emotional aspects of sex, men can enhance their sexual experiences and build deeper connections with their partners.

Kegel exercises, the "stop-start" method, and other body techniques can all help extend and intensify orgasms, while edging is a technique that can build sexual tension and prolong pleasure. It's essential to communicate openly with your partner and prioritize each other's pleasure and desires.

Remember that every individual's sexual journey is unique, and exploring different techniques and approaches to sex can lead to increased pleasure and fulfillment. With an open mind and a willingness to explore new ideas, men can achieve multi-orgasmic sex and embrace sexual empowerment for a lifelong intimate connection with their partner.

It's crucial to practice self-care and prioritize your well-being during any sexual experience. If you're experiencing pain or discomfort, or if you're not enjoying the experience, it's essential to communicate this with your partner and explore new techniques together.

Overall, the art of extended orgasms is about exploring different techniques and approaches to sex, communicating openly with your partner, and prioritizing each other's pleasure and desires. By embracing sexuality as an essential aspect of human connection and fulfillment, men can achieve greater intimacy and lifelong sexual empowerment.

Cheryl Bach

Chapter 5

Achieving Multiple Orgasms

In this chapter, we will explore a step-by-step guide to achieving multiple orgasms as a man, tips for recognizing different types of orgasms and the sensations associated with each one, and different techniques for transitioning between multiple orgasms.

Step-by-Step Guide to Achieving Multiple Orgasms as a Man

Achieving multiple orgasms as a man is a skill that takes practice but can be learned with patience and perseverance.

Here's a step-by-step guide to help you get started:

Build up sexual energy: Building sexual energy is key to achieving multiple orgasms. You can do this by focusing on your breath and becoming more aware of the sensations in your body. You can also use techniques like edging and kegel exercises to build your sexual energy.

Reach your first orgasm: Achieving your first orgasm may take some time but once you do, it can act as a springboard for achieving multiple orgasms. Once you feel close to the point of no return, take a deep breath and slow down or stop stimulation. With practice, you can learn to recognize the sensations associated with this, and build up your sexual energy again without ejaculating.

Relax your body: Relaxing your body helps you build up your sexual energy and prepare your body for multiple orgasms. Take deep breaths, relax your muscles, and focus on the sensations in your body. Try to let go of any performance anxiety or negative thoughts that might interfere with your experience.

Build up your arousal level again: Once you've relaxed, start building up your arousal level again by slowly stimulating yourself or engaging in sexual activity with your partner. Build up your sexual energy gradually, and use different techniques and positions to intensify your arousal. As you start to feel close to the point of no return again, slow down or stop stimulation to prevent ejaculation.

Repeat the process: Once you've achieved your second orgasm, you can repeat the process again to try to achieve multiple orgasms. Remember to take breaks and focus on building up your sexual energy before moving on to the next orgasm.

Tips for Recognizing Different Types of Orgasms

There are several types of orgasms that men can experience, each with different sensations and levels of intensity.

Cheryl Bach

Here are some tips to help you recognize the different types of orgasms:

Prostate Orgasms: Prostate orgasms are achieved by stimulating the prostate gland. They are often described as deeper, more intense orgasms that radiate throughout the body.

Penile Orgasms: Penile orgasms, also known as ejaculatory orgasms, are the most common type of orgasm experienced by men. They usually involve a release of semen and can be accompanied by strong, rhythmic contractions.

Full-Body Orgasms: Full-body orgasms involve intense pleasure that spreads throughout the body. They may be accompanied by shaking or convulsions, and are often described as a spiritual or transcendent experience.

Prolonged Orgasms: Prolonged orgasms can last longer than traditional ejaculatory orgasms and involve a continuous stream of pleasure that doesn't stop after ejaculation. These orgasms are achieved through techniques like edging and can be extremely intense and pleasurable.

Different Techniques for Transitioning Between Multiple Orgasms

There are several techniques that can help you transition between multiple orgasms:

Switching between different types of orgasms: You can transition from one type of orgasm to another by switching the focus of your stimulation. For example, if you've just had a penile orgasm, try focusing on prostate stimulation to achieve a more intense, full-body orgasm.

Changing the intensity and pace of stimulation: By adjusting the level of stimulation and changing the pace of your sexual activity, you can transition between different types of orgasms. For example, starting with slow, gentle stimulation and gradually increasing the intensity to build up to a powerful climax.

Using mental techniques: Mental techniques like visualization and breathing exercises can help you transition between multiple orgasms by laser-focusing on the sensations in your body and making the most of each orgasm. For example, you can try visualizing a wave of pleasure moving through your body or focusing on each individual sensation to reach multiple peaks of pleasure.

Practicing edging: Edging involves bringing yourself close to ejaculation and then holding back, letting the sexual energy build up before starting again. This can help you learn to control your orgasms and build up the necessary sexual energy for multiple orgasms.

Communication with your partner: Communication with your partner is key to achieving multiple orgasms. Let them know what feels good and what doesn't, and work together to find new techniques and approaches that maximize pleasure for both parties.

By practicing these techniques and exploring different types of orgasms, men can achieve multi-orgasmic sex and embrace sexual empowerment for a lifelong intimate connection with their partner. With patience, practice, and open communication, men can unlock new heights of pleasure and deepen their bond with their partner. It's important to remember that everyone's body and sexual preferences are different, and what works for one person may not work for another.

It's also important to prioritize consent and communication in all sexual activity. Always check in with your partner and make sure they are comfortable with the activities you are engaging in. Don't pressure them to try something they aren't interested in, and respect their boundaries at all times.

Cheryl Bach

Chapter 6

Mastering Pleasure and Control

In order to achieve multi-orgasmic sex and enhance pleasure for both partners, it is essential for men to master their own sexual pleasure and control. This involves developing mindfulness, self-awareness, and empathy in sexual encounters, as well as learning techniques for communicating effectively with sexual partners to maximize pleasure and connection.

The Importance of Mindfulness, Self-Awareness, and Empathy in Sexual Encounters

Mindfulness is the practice of being fully present in the moment and aware of one's thoughts, feelings, and sensations. When applied to sexual encounters, mindfulness can help men become more attuned to their own pleasure and the pleasure of their partner. By paying close attention to the physical sensations they are experiencing and the emotional connection they are building with their partner, men can enhance their sexual experiences and achieve greater levels of pleasure.

Self-awareness is the process of introspection and reflection on one's own thoughts, emotions, and behavior. In the context of multi-orgasmic sex, self-awareness can help men identify their own sexual triggers, preferences, and limitations. This knowledge can be used to tailor sexual experiences to maximize pleasure and minimize discomfort or pain. Self-awareness can also help men become more comfortable with their own bodies and desires, reducing feelings of shame or inadequacy that can interfere with sexual pleasure.

Empathy is the ability to understand and share the emotions and perspectives of others. In sexual encounters, empathy can help men attune to their partner's needs and desires, fostering a sense of emotional connection and deepening intimacy. By being open to their partner's feedback and reactions, men can adjust their own behavior to better meet their partner's needs and enhance mutual pleasure.

Techniques for Communicating Effectively with Sexual Partners to Maximize Pleasure and Connection

Effective communication is another key component of mastering pleasure and control in the context of multi-orgasmic sex. Communication involves not only expressing one's own desires and needs, but also listening actively to one's partner and responding in ways that promote mutual pleasure.

Here are some techniques that can help men communicate more effectively in sexual encounters:

Use non-verbal communication: Sometimes words can get in the way of effective communication. Using non-verbal cues like moans, gasps, and body movements can convey pleasure and communicate what feels good in the moment.

Ask for feedback: Don't assume that you know what your partner wants or needs. Instead, ask for feedback throughout the encounter. For example, "Does this feel good?" or "How can I make you feel even better?"

Share your fantasies: Sharing your sexual fantasies with your partner can help open up new avenues of pleasure and deepen intimacy. It's important to do this in a way that is respectful of your partner's boundaries and comfort level, and to listen to their fantasies as well.

Practice active listening: Active listening involves truly paying attention to your partner and understanding their perspective. This means being present in the moment, avoiding distracting thoughts or behaviors, and paraphrasing what your partner has said to ensure that you have understood them correctly.

Use "I" statements: When expressing your own desires or needs, try to use "I" statements rather than "you" statements. For example, instead of saying "You never do X," say "I really like it when we do X together."

By developing mindfulness, self-awareness, empathy, and effective communication skills, men can master their own pleasure and control and achieve multi-orgasmic sex. These techniques can also lead to a deeper sense of intimacy and connection with sexual partners, enhancing overall sexual fulfillment and satisfaction.

Tools and Strategies for Mastering Pleasure and Control

Another important aspect of mastering pleasure and control in multi-orgasmic sex is developing a strong sense of sexual confidence. Sexual confidence involves feeling comfortable and secure in one's own sexual abilities, preferences, and desires, and being able to communicate those effectively with a partner.

To develop sexual confidence, men can try the following strategies:

Explore your own body: Take the time to explore your own body and become familiar with what feels pleasurable and what doesn't. This can involve solo experimentation or exploration with a partner.

Learn about sex: Read books or articles, watch videos, or attend workshops or classes that provide information on different sexual techniques and approaches. Having knowledge about sex can boost confidence and reduce anxiety or uncertainty.

Surround yourself with positive influences: Seek out friends, partners, or communities that are accepting of diverse sexual experiences and encourage open communication about pleasure and desire. Being around positive influences can help alleviate shame or anxiety about sexual experiences, allowing for greater comfort and confidence in exploring sexuality.

Practice self-acceptance: Acceptance of one's own body, desires, and preferences is crucial for developing sexual confidence. Recognize that everyone has different sexual needs and desires, and embrace your own uniqueness without judgment.

Take things slow: Rushing into sexual experiences or focusing solely on orgasm as the end goal can lead to anxiety or pressure, which can inhibit pleasure and confidence. Instead, focus on building intimacy and connection with a partner, taking time to explore and experiment without judgment or expectations.

By combining mindfulness, self-awareness, empathy, effective communication, and sexual confidence, men can develop the tools and strategies necessary to master pleasure and control in multi-orgasmic sex. These skills can lead to deeper levels of intimacy, trust, and connection with sexual partners, leading to greater overall sexual fulfillment and satisfaction.

Of course, it's important to remember that sexual experiences are complex and multifaceted, influenced by a variety of factors such as physical health, emotional wellbeing, and relationship dynamics. However, by focusing on the aforementioned tools and strategies, men can work towards improving their own sexual experiences and enhancing overall sexual well-being.

Chapter 7

Sexual Empowerment and Fulfilment for Lifelong Wellness

Embracing multi-orgasmic sex can lead to an unparalleled sense of sexual empowerment for men. By cultivating mindfulness, self-awareness, empathy, and effective communication skills, men can achieve greater control over their own pleasure, satisfaction, and overall well-being.

To fully embrace multi-orgasmic sex, it's important to view sexuality as an essential component of overall health and wellness. This means developing lifelong practices that prioritize sexual fulfillment and pleasure, while also maintaining safe, respectful, and responsible sexual practices.

Strategies for Integrating Multi-Orgasmic Sex into Lifelong Sexual Wellness Practices

One key strategy for integrating multi-orgasmic sex into lifelong sexual wellness practices is focused on building a solid foundation of sexual knowledge and understanding. This includes learning about one's own body, desires, and preferences, as well as exploring different sexual techniques and approaches with a partner. Knowledge and understanding can boost confidence, reduce anxiety and uncertainty, and promote a deeper sense of intimacy and connection with sexual partners.

Another key strategy for embracing multi-orgasmic sex is to prioritize individual sexuality and pleasure. This means developing a strong sense of self-awareness and comfort with one's own sexual desires and preferences, without judgment or shame. It also means being willing to communicate openly and honestly with a partner about one's own needs and desires, while also respecting their boundaries and preferences.

Exploring How Embracing Multi-Orgasmic Sex Can Lead to Sexual Empowerment for Men

In addition to individual sexuality, embracing multi-orgasmic sex also involves prioritizing the intimate connection and mutual pleasure with a partner. Cultivating effective communication skills, such as active listening, nonverbal cues, and "I" statements, can facilitate communication and understanding between partners, leading to deeper levels of intimacy and pleasure.

Finally, embracing multi-orgasmic sex requires embracing positive and respectful attitudes towards ourselves and others. This means avoiding harmful attitudes or behaviors that perpetuate toxic masculinity, such as objectification, dominance, or aggression. Instead, it means embracing respectful, consensual, and empathetic approaches to sexual experiences that prioritize the well-being and pleasure of all involved.

Incorporating these strategies into lifelong sexual wellness practices can lead to a greater sense of sexual empowerment and fulfillment for men. By understanding and embracing our own sexuality, communicating openly and honestly with partners, and prioritizing mutual pleasure and respect, we can achieve multi-orgasmic sex and a deeper sense of connection and intimacy with our partners.

Positive Approaches to Individual Sexuality and Fulfilling Intimate Connection with One's Partner

To fully embrace multi-orgasmic sex and sexual empowerment, it's important to approach sexuality with an open mind and willingness to learn and grow. This means recognizing that sexuality is an ever-evolving and complex aspect of human experience, and that there is always room for exploration and discovery.

Men can engage in practices such as mindfulness, meditation, and physical exercise to cultivate self-awareness, increase relaxation, and improve overall health and well-being. These practices can help create more fertile ground for sexual exploration and fulfillment, while also promoting mental and emotional wellness.

In addition to these practices, men can also prioritize sexual health by getting regular STI testing, practicing safe sex, and seeking medical assistance when necessary. Doing so not only protects one's own well-being but also promotes a culture of sexual responsibility and respect.

Ultimately, embracing multi-orgasmic sex and sexual empowerment requires a commitment to self-improvement, mutual respect, and open communication. By cultivating a positive attitude towards sexuality and prioritizing pleasure and connection with our partners, we can achieve a lifetime of sexual fulfillment, intimacy, and well-being.

Conclusion

Overview of Key Takeaways from the Guide

Through the course of this guide, we have explored various techniques, strategies, and approaches to help men achieve multi-orgasmic sex, master pleasure, and embrace sexual empowerment for lifelong fulfillment and intimate connection.

Here's a quick overview of the key takeaways and insights shared in this guide:

- Multi-orgasmic sex is achievable by men, with practice, patience, and the right mindset.

- Mindfulness, relaxation, and focused breathing can help control ejaculation and enhance sexual pleasure.

- Building a strong foundation of sexual knowledge and understanding can boost confidence, reduce anxiety, and promote deeper intimacy and connection with sexual partners.

- Effective communication skills, such as active listening, nonverbal cues, and "I" statements, can facilitate communication and understanding between partners, leading to deeper levels of intimacy and pleasure.

- Embracing positive attitudes and rejecting toxic masculinity can lead to respectful, consensual, and empathetic approaches to sexual experiences.

- Lifelong sexual exploration and fulfillment requires a commitment to self-improvement, mutual respect, and open communication.

Encouragement towards Lifelong Sexual Exploration, Empowerment, and Fulfillment as a Man.

As a man, it's important to approach sexuality with an open mind and a willingness to learn and grow. By developing strategies for achieving multi-orgasmic sex, cultivating self-awareness and relaxation practices, building a strong foundation of sexual knowledge and understanding, and embracing positive attitudes and healthy practices, men can achieve sexual empowerment for lifelong fulfillment and intimate connection.

It's important to remember that sexuality is a personal experience that is ever-evolving and unique to each individual. This guide should be viewed as a starting point for exploration and discovery, rather than a definitive set of instructions or rules. The key is to approach sexuality with an open mind, a willingness to experiment and explore, and a focus on pleasure and connection.

It's also important to prioritize sexual health and safety. Men should get regular STI testing, practice safe sex, and seek medical assistance when necessary. By protecting their own well-being, men can promote a culture of sexual responsibility and respect.

In conclusion, this guide is a comprehensive resource for men to achieve multi-orgasmic sex, master pleasure, and embrace sexual empowerment for lifelong fulfillment and intimate connection. By incorporating the strategies and techniques shared in this guide into everyday sexual wellbeing practices, men can achieve a deeper sense of intimacy and pleasure with their partners, while also promoting mental, emotional, and physical well-being. So go forth, explore your sexuality, and embrace the joys of multi-orgasmic sex for a lifetime of sexual fulfillment and intimate connection.